Managed Health Care Guide for Caseworkers and Foster Parents

Ellen Sittenfeld Battistelli

CWLA Press • Washington, DC

The Child Welfare League of America expresses its gratitude to the Robert Wood Johnson Foundation for its generous support in this effort and its ongoing committment to the well-being of children in out-of-home care.

CWLA Press is an imprint of the Child Welfare League of America.

CHILD WELFARE LEAGUE OF AMERICA, INC.
440 First Street, NW, Third Floor, Washington, DC 20001-2085
Email: books@cwla.org

CURRENT PRINTING (last digit)
10 9 8 7 6 5 4 3 2 1

Cover design by Sarah Knipschild
Text design by Eve Malakoff-Klein

Printed in the United States of America

Library of Congress Cataloging-in-Publication Data
Battistelli, Ellen Sittenfeld.
    Managed health care guide for caseworkers and foster parents / by Ellen Sittenfeld Battistelli
        p.   cm.
    ISBN 0–87868–682–7 (pbk.)
    1. Foster children--Medical care--United States.   2. Managed care plans (Medical care)--United States.   I. Title.
RJ102.B37   1997
362.1'04258--dc21   97–19976

For Molly, Joey, and Becky

who show the need for, the right to, and the rewards of all children having good health care.

Contents

Preface

This *Managed Care Guide for Caseworkers and Foster Parents* is designed to answer the many questions that foster parents and caseworkers have about managed health care and its impact on children in foster care. Over the last several years, the health needs of children in care have increased greatly in both number and complexity. At the same time, there have been significant changes in the way that health care services are delivered and financed, with a trend toward the use of managed care to serve Medicaid-eligible children in general and children in foster care in particular. What will managed care mean for children in foster care? Will managed care be responsive to the comprehensive health care needs of children in care? How can foster parents and caseworkers make the most of managed care in behalf of these children?

This guide, supported by a grant from the Robert Wood Johnson Foundation, provides foster parents and caseworkers with an easy-to-read resource regarding managed care, and with the information they need to ensure that managed care works effectively for the children for whom they are responsible. Managed care *can* work for children in foster care, but it will work best when foster parents and caseworkers understand the managed care system and know how to intervene in behalf of the children in their care.

Introduction

The health care system in the United States is rapidly changing. At one time, individuals with health insurance, including Medicaid, could choose a doctor, receive health care services, and have their insurance pay most or all of the cost. Today, more and more people with health insurance, including Medicaid, are being required to enroll in "managed care plans," which place controls on their choice of health care providers, the services they can receive, and the costs of those services. In many communities, managed care is an option for children in care; in others, children in care are being required to obtain their health care through managed care organizations.

Managed care is both loved and hated. When managed care works well for children, the provision of health care is well coordinated; a full range of prevention and treatment services is available; care is provided by well-qualified doctors and other health care providers who understand the needs of children; and the doctor-patient relationship is a positive experience.

When managed care does not work well for children, all of the services children need—especially specialized pediatric health, mental health, and developmental services—may not be available; caregivers may have difficulty scheduling appointments for health care services; and the services provided may not be of a high quality or may be inappropriate.

Quality health care for children in care is essential. Study after study has shown that children in care have more health problems than any other group in the United States. Often, their problems are the result of the abuse and neglect that brought them into care. Sometimes, their problems intensify as a result of their stay in foster care, as they try to cope with separation from their biological families and uncertainty about what will happen to them.

In the current health care environment, foster parents and caseworkers can help meet the health needs of children in care by:

- understanding how managed care works and how to use managed care effectively in behalf of the children in their care;

- knowing how to advocate for the children in their care when managed care fails to respond to the needs of those children; and

- actively participating in all aspects of the children's health care.

This *Managed Health Care Guide for Caseworkers and Foster Parents* provides caregivers with the information they need to accomplish these tasks. Chapter 1, *The Health Care Needs of Children in Foster Care*, provides an overview of the physical, emotional, and developmental health care needs of children in care. It lists some of the health problems that children in care often have and explains how to obtain as much information as possible about children's health histories.

Chapter 2, *Understanding the Health Care System*, describes the basic ways that health care has been provided to children in care, as well as recent changes arising from the implementation of managed care. It explains Medicaid and provides a general outline of managed care.

Chapter 3, *Using Managed Care Services*, focuses on the "nuts and bolts" of using a managed care plan, including choosing a plan and a primary care physician, making appointments, and obtaining referrals.

Chapter 4, *Advocating for Children*, explains how and where to get help, both inside and outside the managed care plan.

Chapter 5, *Managed Care Questions and Answers*, answers some of the most frequently asked questions about managed care. It also provides concrete examples of difficulties that may arise and suggests actions that foster parents and caseworkers might take in response.

Appendix A lists symptoms of medical, mental health, and developmental problems often seen in children in care; *Appendix B* provides a glossary of commonly used managed care terms; and *Appendix C* provides a sample immunization schedule.

Chapter One

The Health Care Needs of Children in Foster Care

Most children who enter foster care have one or more health problems that need immediate attention. These problems may be physical, emotional, or developmental. Some are problems the children were born with; others may have developed over time. Some may have been partially treated, others not treated at all, and still others not even diagnosed. While all children need preventive and primary care (immunizations, well-baby and well-child check-ups, and screening for basic problems), many children in foster care have never received these health care services.

The health problems of children entering care may be the result of many factors. For some children, their mothers' use of tobacco, alcohol, and/or drugs during pregnancy may have caused physical and developmental problems. Many were exposed in their own homes to lead and other unhealthy conditions. Other children may suffer from neglect. They may not have had enough food, seen a doctor regularly, had their immunizations when they should, or been given enough attention or stimulation to develop socially, emotionally, or cognitively as healthy children do.

Children in foster care have often been abused physically, emotionally, or sexually; these experiences frequently result in serious health problems that require long-term treatment. Adolescents entering care may bring with them alcohol and/or drug problems of their own, as well as health issues related to sexual activity, including the possibility of pregnancy and sexually transmitted diseases. Finally, a growing number of children entering care are HIV positive, and will need a range of long-term health care services.

The Importance of Comprehensive Health Care

Foster care provides an opportunity for children entering care to have their health care needs comprehensively addressed. While in care, children can receive the primary and preventive health care services they need, including up-to-date immunizations; screening and diagnostic services to identify their health care needs; treatment services for their physical health, mental health, and developmental needs; and specialized services as necessary. Foster care also provides an opportunity for biological parents to learn more about their children's health care needs and how to use the health care system and other community services (e.g., Head Start, special education) to meet those needs.

A Shared Responsibility

Foster parents and caseworkers are important resources for children as well as their biological parents. The foster parents' day-to-day contact with the children provides an opportunity to observe problems the children may be having and to work closely with the caseworkers to meet the children's needs. The caseworkers' ongoing contact with the children's biological parents provides an opportunity to obtain important health background information and to work with them to understand and respond to their children's health care needs. Because most children return home to their parents, obtaining this information and teaching parents these skills will be critical to the children's ongoing health and well-being.

Obtaining a Health History

Most children who enter foster care do not have complete health care records, nor do they have a single doctor who knows them well. Some information, however, is likely to be available. The caseworker should obtain as much information as possible about the child's health history. This information will provide the foster parents with a better understanding of the child's needs and will provide the doctor and other health care providers who work with the child with important background information.

The Role of the Caseworker

There are several steps the caseworker can take to obtain as comprehensive a health history for the child as possible.

1. The caseworker should obtain health information from the child's biological parents.
The caseworker should make every effort to learn about the child's health background from the child's parents. This information should include:

- The child's known medical problems, including drug allergies, serious accidents or injuries, surgeries, hospitalizations, and seizures;

- The types of immunizations the child has received and the dates of those immunizations;

- Any medications the child is taking (the name, the dose, when to administer it, and the reason it is being taken);

- Any physical, mental health, or developmental problems the parent has observed or has concerns about;

- The names of doctors and other health care providers that the child has seen, including the name of the hospital where the child was born; and

- Any other available relevant health information.

2. The caseworker should obtain copies of all available health care records concerning the child.

The caseworker should ask the biological parents to authorize the release of health care information on their child, and should request health care records from all doctors and health care providers that the parents can identify.

3. The caseworker should identify the agency's health care coordinator for the foster parents.
Some child welfare agencies have an individual on staff who coordinates health services for children in foster care and who is responsible for obtaining the child's background health information. The caseworker should provide the foster parents with the coordinator's name, office hours, and telephone number.

4. The caseworker should schedule and follow up on an initial health screening for the child.
All children entering care should have an initial health evaluation, before placement, if possible, but in any event, no later than 24 hours following placement. This initial evaluation should be used to identify any health problems that might require immediate attention or affect the placement chosen.

5. The caseworker should schedule a complete health assessment for the child.
All children entering care should have a complete health assessment within 30 days of placement. The assessment should identify any health problems that require immediate treatment and any problems that require ongoing health care services. The caseworker should ensure that the assessment takes place and that the doctor who does the assessment provides a written report (including recommendations for further treatment and care) to the child welfare agency and to the foster parents.

6. The caseworker should communicate with the foster parents about the child's health status and health care needs.
The caseworker should meet with the foster parents to review what has been learned about the child's health status and health care needs from the discussion with the child's biological parents, the review of the health care records, and the screening assessment. This discussion with the foster parents should result in a health care plan for the child that includes:

- what follow-up care is needed;

- what kind of health care services the child needs and why;

- what kind of doctors or health care providers the child needs to see and how to make the appointment;

- what kind of medication the child should take and why;

- what signs or symptoms to look for (to know when to a contact a doctor); and

- what types of precautions to take to safeguard the child's health.

7. The caseworker should communicate with the foster parents about the responsibilities that they and the child welfare agency have.
The caseworker should clarify for the foster parents that they are responsible for observing the child's health and notifying the agency of any problems they observe or have concerns about, taking the child to see doctors and other health care providers, and providing the agency with follow-up reports on the child's health care needs and services received. States vary in their statements of policy and practice regarding consent for medical care. Most often, the child welfare agency, because it has legal custody of the child, has the final responsibility for the child's health care. Some states, however, require the involvement of the court or the child's biological parents when consent to certain types of care or treatment is needed.

The Role of the Foster Parents

1. The foster parents should talk with the caseworker about the child's health status and health care needs.
The foster parents should meet with the caseworker to talk about the child's health status and health care needs, and should ask the caseworker to review the information obtained from the child's biological parents, the health care records, and the health assessment.

2. The foster parents should develop with the caseworker a health care plan for the child.

The foster parents should take part in developing a plan that addresses the child's current and future health care needs. The foster parents should make sure they understand:

- the child's immediate and long-term health care needs;

- the types of doctors or health care providers the child needs to see;

- the medications the child should take;

- the precautions that should be taken to safeguard the child's health at home and at school (if the child is school age), as well as to safeguard the health of others.

Identifying Other Health Care Problems

Foster parents can play an important role in identifying other health care problems that the children in their care may have. The foster parents see the child every day in different situations and are likely to be the first to notice that a problem exists. While the foster parents cannot diagnose a health condition or problem, they can make note of possible problems and notify both the caseworker and the child's doctor or other health care provider.

Foster parents normally are in the best position to observe warning signs about physical and/or emotional problems that have not yet been identified. They can help doctors and health care providers identify problems by noticing behaviors such as:

- hiding or hoarding food;

- prolonged crying;

- withdrawn behavior;

- aggressive behavior toward others or toward self, including self-mutilation;

- sudden changes in behavior;

- excessive eating or drinking;

- poor appetite or change in appetite;

- bulimia/anorexia;

- sexualized behavior;

- hyperactive behavior;
- sleep disturbances;
- bedwetting;
- temper tantrums;
- stealing;
- lying;
- nervousness;
- excessive daydreaming;
- hearing voices;
- delusional thinking (beliefs not based in reality);
- unusual habits or movements; or
- unusual responses to common experiences or events.

Of course, it is equally important that foster parents look for positive signs that the child in their care is healthy and growing normally. Some of the positive indicators are:

- height and weight within normal range for age;
- acts in a way that is typical of age;
- acts as if he/she is feeling good;
- has fewer sick days over time in the foster care home; and
- lets foster parents know when he/she isn't feeling well.

Appendix A lists the symptoms of health, mental health, and developmental problems that often affect children in foster care. Foster parents and caseworkers should be aware of these potential problems and discuss any concerns they have with the child's caseworker, or doctor or other health care provider.

Chapter Two

Understanding the Health Care System

Once the health care problems and needs of the children in their care are identified, the foster parents and caseworkers must locate and use the necessary health care services, and obtain payment for those services. For children in foster care, the federal Medicaid program is the primary funder of health care services. Increasingly, the Medicaid program is turning to managed care to provide and pay for health care services for children in foster care. Caseworkers and foster parents need a basic understanding of the Medicaid program and the way that Medicaid and managed care are now attempting to work together.

The Medicaid Program

Medicaid is a joint federal-state government program that funds health care services for individuals who are poor, very sick, or elderly. It is, in effect, health insurance for certain individuals. Most children in foster care are eligible for Medicaid and can obtain services through the program at no cost to the foster family or the agency responsible for them. Under Medicaid, children in foster care can obtain primary and preventive health care, such as immunizations, treatment for medical problems, mental health care services, and, in some areas, developmental services.

The Importance of the Medicaid Card

When a child enters foster care, the caseworker must complete the paperwork necessary to obtain a Medicaid card for the child. The card is proof of coverage through Medicaid. It gives the doctor or other health care provider the information needed to bill Medicaid for the services provided. Foster parents should receive a Medicaid card for each child in their care. The Medicaid card is the key to obtaining needed health care services.

Medicaid Services

Under federal law, children covered by Medicaid (including children in foster care) are entitled to the following services:

1. *Regular assessments and full examinations of the child's medical, developmental, vision, hearing, dental, and mental health, including (at specific ages):*

- height, weight, and head size measurements;

- blood pressure screening;

- vision and hearing tests;

- checks of the heart and lungs;

- genital examination;

- observation of the child's movements; and

- discussion with the foster parents or caregivers about the child's eating, sleeping, daily activities, and relationships with friends and family.

2. *Regular health care screenings (at specific ages) for:*

- tuberculosis (a highly contagious lung disease that can be fatal if not properly treated);

- sickle cell anemia (an inherited blood disorder most commonly found in persons of African American ancestry);

- anemia (a condition in which low levels of iron in the blood cause weakness and tiredness); and

- HIV (the virus that causes AIDS). A child may be born HIV positive if his or her mother was infected with the virus, or may acquire the virus through intravenous drug use or unprotected sex.

3. *Immunizations to protect them from several serious infectious diseases, including chicken pox, polio, measles, mumps, and tetanus.*

4. *Health education.*
Children should be taught how to keep themselves healthy—how to eat right, brush their teeth, get enough sleep, not take drugs, abstain from sex or protect themselves from pregnancy and sexually transmitted diseases.

5. *Referrals and follow-up treatment to correct or remedy identified problems.*
Children covered by Medicaid are entitled to receive the services needed to determine the existence of a possible illness or condition, as well as the care and services needed to improve or cure the condition.

Medicaid Providers

In the past, each state's Medicaid program "enrolled" doctors and other health care providers in its program. These providers agreed to see Medicaid-covered individuals and agreed to accept whatever Medicaid paid for the service. Medicaid-covered individuals were free to see any doctor or health care provider who agreed to accept Medicaid payments for their services. The charge for the service was based on a "fee-for-service" approach, that is, the doctor provided the health care service to the patient and then billed the Medicaid program a fee for that service. Under this system, doctors made the decisions about what services were needed and how many times they needed to see patients. Although this system remains in effect in some places, in many states and communities the Medicaid program is changing from a fee-for-service approach to a managed care system.

Managed Care

Managed care is a way of providing and paying for health care services that developed because of concerns that the cost of providing health care had become too great. Managed care tries to

> ### Caseworker/Foster Parent Tip
>
> The goals of managed care are to cut health care costs and improve health care quality. MCOs want to control costs and often will build in incentives to make this happen. In some MCO arrangements, doctors may make more money if they do not refer a child for tests or specialty care. While the MCOs argue that such arrangements prevent referrals for unnecessary services, they also can result in the child not getting to the right doctor for the right treatment at the right time. As a foster parent or caseworker, you must commit yourself to fighting for quality and to making sure that the child in your care receives all necessary services.

control the costs of health care by setting limits—limits on which doctors or health care providers a patient may see, limits on the kinds of services the insurance company will pay for, limits on the number of services that a patient may receive, and limits on how much the insurer will pay for the services provided. Because managed care organizations (MCO), as insurers, are financially responsible for the care of those who become ill, they do have a vested interest in helping patients to get healthy and stay healthy. The hope is that managed care will achieve the same or better health outcomes as traditional fee-for-service plans do, but at less cost.

How Managed Care Works

The key players in managed care are called *managed care organizations* or MCOs.* MCOs pay for health care services; decide who gets services, what services can be obtained, and for how long services will be provided; and enter into contracts with doctors and other health care providers to provide services under specific rules. MCOs work to limit the costs of health care by, for example, monitoring doctors and other health care providers to see how efficiently they treat patients; limiting the number of tests that

---

* *Appendix B provides a glossary of key terms.*

health care providers can order or perform; limiting the use of specialists, whose services tend to be expensive; and requiring documentation of need before expensive treatments are provided.

The way that managed care works can be illustrated best by comparing the traditional Medicaid fee-for-service approach with the managed care approach currently being implemented by Medicaid, as shown in the chart on the next page.

The Benefits of Managed Care

Those who believe that managed care represents a sound approach to health care say that managed care can reduce costs and at the same time:

- provide appropriate and efficient services;
- improve recordkeeping and accountability;
- stop unnecessary and inappropriate medical tests and procedures;
- offer preventive and primary health care to catch and treat illness early;
- offer health education;
- offer comprehensive and coordinated care;
- provide case management;
- increase accessibility through convenient service locations and office hours;
- increase accessibility by offering medical assistance by telephone; and
- reduce the use of hospital emergency rooms by reserving their use for life-threatening emergencies.

The Drawbacks of Managed Care

Those who do not believe that managed care is a good approach to health care say that managed care:

- keeps patients from getting the specialized services they need, including the services of pediatric specialists;

Fee for Service and Managed Care: A Comparison

Fee for Service	Managed Care
Patients choose their own doctor and hospital (provided they accept Medicaid patients).	Patients go only to doctors and hospitals the MCO has signed up as part of the managed care network.
Patients get care when, where and how they want—doctor's office, clinic, emergency room (provided they accept Medicaid-covered individuals).	Patients get care where, when, and how the MCO says.
Patients get as much care as the doctor decides.	Patients get as much care as the gatekeeper and MCO decide.
Doctors/other providers are paid after they provide a service.	Doctors/other providers are paid a fixed amount per year, whether or not they provide any care and regardless of the type and amount of care they provide.
Patients receive as many services as they and the doctors decide—perhaps too many (that is, they may get services they don't really need).	Patients may receive only a limited number of services—perhaps too few services (that is, they may not get necessary services).
Patients can change doctors anytime.	Patients may change doctors according to the rules of the plan and/or the Medicaid contract.

- limits the provision of health care services by providing doctors and other health care providers with incentives not to provide services or to make referrals for services;

- limits choice of doctors and other health care providers;

- results in medical decisions being made by doctors, often within limits set by the MCOs;

- pushes additional patients into doctors' offices and away from community-based clinics and other programs;

- creates bureaucratic obstacles to obtaining specialized care;

- uses providers who are far away from or inaccessible to patients; and

- leads to delays in obtaining appointments.

Managed Care's Effect on Children in Foster Care

Because the use of managed care in Medicaid is relatively new for children in foster care, it is not clear what the effects of managed care will be. How will MCOs look at children in foster care? Will children in foster care be treated like all other children or will MCOs recognize that they have many more and much more serious health problems than their peers in the general population? Chapters 3 and 4 present key concepts to help caseworkers and foster parents make managed care work for the children in their care.

Chapter Three

Using Managed Care Services

When children in foster care are enrolled in a managed care plan, their foster parents and caseworkers must understand how to use the system effectively to meet their needs. This chapter explains some of the key steps in effectively using managed care. Chapter 5 provides answers to commonly asked questions concerning the use of managed care.

Enrolling in a Managed Care Plan

If a child in foster care will be receiving health care through a managed care organization, one of two events will happen:

- The child welfare agency will enroll the child in a plan (the agency may have only one plan to use or may have a choice of plans); or

- The child welfare agency will allow the foster parents to choose the managed care plan for the child.

If a choice of plans is permitted, the foster parents and caseworker should evaluate the health care provider network, provider accessibility, services covered, and quality of services in deciding which plan is best for the child.

Evaluating the Provider Network

- Does the plan have pediatricians and pediatric specialists in its provider network?

- Do the doctors and other health care providers have experience treating children in foster care?

- Does the plan offer specialists in areas in which the child has needs? For example, does the plan have doctors specializing in children's allergies or heart problems?

- Can the agency/foster parents choose the child's doctor?

- How easy is it to change the child's doctor?

- What hospitals are in the network? Is the plan affiliated with a children's hospital (if available) rather than a general hospital with a pediatric unit?

Evaluating Provider Accessibility

- Are the providers in a location convenient to the foster home? To public transportation?

- What are the provider's hours? Are services provided in the evenings and on weekends?

- How long does it take to get an appointment to see a doctor?

- Does the provider help with transportation if needed?

- Do the doctors and staff speak the child's and/or foster parents' language?

- Does the plan have a 24-hour telephone advice line that provides medical information and first-aid advice?

Evaluating the Service Coverage

- What pediatric services does the plan cover?

- What pediatric services does the plan exclude?

- Does the plan have specialized mental health care services for children?

- Does the plan offer developmental services?

- Does the plan cover occupational therapy, physical therapy, or speech therapy?
- Does the plan offer dental services?
- Does the plan pay for hearing aids, eyeglasses, and other medical equipment (wheelchairs, splints, crutches, respiratory equipment, bed-wetting alarms, etc.)?
- Does the plan offer home health care services?
- Does the plan offer visiting nurse care?

Evaluating the Quality of Services

- If the foster parents are not satisfied with the quality of care being provided to the child, what can they do?
- How does the plan review the quality of care its providers give?
- Are the plan's grievance and appeal procedures easy to understand?
- What is the MCO's history related to appeals?

> ### *Caseworker/Foster Parent Tip*
> Managed care organizations usually offer written materials about their plans, including descriptions of the plans and their benefits, a list of the doctors and other health care providers who provide services, written grievance and appeal procedures, and instructions on how to get additional information. Foster parents and caseworkers can ask the MCO or the state Medicaid office to send them a copy of all written materials on the plan.

- What is the accountability of the MCO for the outcome of its decisions?
- How and how often can the child change an MCO plan?

The Primary Care Physician

Choosing a Primary Care Physician

Once a plan is selected, the agency or foster parent will be asked to select a primary care physician or PCP. The PCP provides the

---
Caseworker/Foster Parent Tip

If none of the possible PCPs are familiar, check with other foster parents who have children enrolled in the plan to find out who they prefer and work best with. Many states have foster parent associations that can provide information on which plans work best for children in care and which do not.
---

child with health exams and immunizations, takes care of illnesses and injuries, makes referrals to specialists when necessary, and coordinates all health services the child needs. He or she is the "gatekeeper" who decides what services the child needs and who should provide those services. MCOs usually will not pay for additional health care services unless the PCP preapproves them.

The MCO usually provides a list of doctors from which the foster parents or caseworker can select the child's PCP. In choosing the PCP, the following factors should be considered:

- Are any pediatricians listed as possible PCPs? (It is usually best to select as the PCP a doctor specifically trained and experienced in children's health care.)

- Are any of the possible PCPs experienced in treating children in foster care?

- Does the child have an ongoing relationship with any of the possible PCPs?

- Do the foster parents already know any of the possible PCPs? If so, are there doctors with whom the foster parents will feel comfortable and can talk easily?

The PCP should be able and willing to work with the foster parents. A good relationship with the PCP begins with the first visit.

Preparing for the First Visit

Prior to the first visit, the caseworker should give to the foster parents or send directly to the PCP:

- a copy of the child's health records, including any health history information and immunization records; and

- current infor-
mation on the
child's medi-
cal, emotional,
or develop-
mental status

> ### *Caseworker/Foster Parent Tip*
> The first visit to the doctor should not
> be delayed even if the child's health
> records are not yet available.

(e.g., a copy of a recent psychological evaluation).

When making the first appointment with the PCP, the foster parents should explain that it will be the child's first visit, that the child is in foster care, and that there are a number of questions that the foster parents will want to ask the doctor. The foster parents should ask to have extra time scheduled for the appointment. It should take the PCP at least 30 minutes to review the child's history, examine the child, and talk with the foster parents.

The First Visit

In addition to the information sent to the PCP in advance of the first visit, on the first visit the foster parents should bring:

- the child's Medicaid card and any other identification card issued by the MCO;

- a list of medications the child takes; and

- a list of questions for the doctor (it may be hard to remember everything that needs to be discussed).

The foster parents should let the doctor know that they want to talk with him or her about the child's needs and should be ready to discuss any concerns about the child's growth and development, illnesses, mood, behavior, eating and sleeping patterns, and past, current, and future health care needs.

The foster parents should ask the doctor questions and get his or her guidance on any concerns they may have. If the doctor's response is complicated and not easy to understand, they should ask again and continue to ask until they clearly understand:

- what the child's health problems are;

- what the recommended treatment is (who needs to see the child, when, how often, for what services);

> ### Caseworker/Foster Parent Tip
> If the doctor talks in technical language and you don't understand what is being said, ask if someone else who works with the doctor will talk further with you. It is the doctor's responsibility to clearly explain what is happening—it is NOT your fault for not understanding. You might also ask to have important information written down or borrow a tape recorder to record the doctor's explanations.

• what medications, if any, are needed, and where they can be obtained;

• what the instructions for the care of the child at home (and at school if the child is school-age) are; and

• what each medication does and its possible side effects or interactions.

Follow-Up Appointments with the PCP or Specialists

At each visit with the PCP, the foster parents should come prepared to discuss the child's needs and any concerns that they have. Maintaining open communication with the PCP is essential to formulating a good plan for the child.

If the child needs a specialist, the foster parents should work with the pediatrician to choose a provider who has experience working with children and, when possible, with children in foster care. They should ask the PCP to explain why the child needs to see a specialist and what information the specialist will need at the first visit. It is important that the child not see a specialist without the PCP's approval. Without that approval, the foster parents may have to pay for the specialist's services.

> ### Caseworker/Foster Parent Tip
> When making appointments with the PCP, explain the purpose of the visit: a checkup, follow-up, assessment, immediate problem, or urgent problem.

Chapter Four

Advocating for Children

To make sure that children in foster care receive the health care services they need, the foster parents and caseworker must work as a team with the children's doctors and other health care providers. To be effective members of this team, the foster parents and caseworker must take on certain responsibilities; they also have the right to expect certain benefits for the children for whom they are responsible.

Rights and Responsibilities

Responsibilities of the Foster Parents

The foster parents are responsible for:

- understanding how managed care plans work and how to use a managed care plan;
- asking for and carefully reading the managed care plan's written policies;
- asking questions and insisting on answers;
- understanding the services the child can receive;
- making sure that all available health information is provided to the health care providers;

- being available to the health care providers on a timely basis to discuss the child's status and their concerns about his/her health or well-being;

- participating in decisions about the child's health care;

- making certain that the child gets to all scheduled health care appointments;

- making certain that the child receives appropriate health care when he/she is ill;

- making certain that the child takes prescribed medication;

- understanding the child's health status and providing information about the child's health to the health care provider and to the caseworker;

- communicating to the health care provider and the caseworker the child's progress or problems; and

- providing information on the child's health status and needs when the child leaves the foster home to return home or to move to another foster care placement.

Responsibilities of the Caseworker

The caseworker is responsible for:

- understanding managed care;

- asking for and carefully reading the managed care plan's written policies;

- ensuring that foster parents receive the managed care plan's written policies and assisting them in understanding those policies;

- ensuring that the child's enrollment forms are completed in a timely way;

- asking questions and insisting on answers;

- understanding the services the child can receive, and assisting the foster parents in understanding those services;

- ensuring that all available health information is provided to the health care providers;

- being available to the health care providers on a timely basis to discuss the child's status and concerns about his/her health or well-being;

- communicating with the foster parents about the child's health care status and needs and the decisions that need to be made about the child's health care;

- assisting the foster parents, as needed, in getting the child to all scheduled health care appointments;

- making certain that the child receives appropriate health care when he/she is ill;

- understanding the child's medication needs and discussing the child's medication with the foster parents;

- understanding the child's health status and needs by communicating with the foster parents and the health care provider when and if needed;

- communicating regularly with the foster parents about the child's health progress;

- ensuring that, should the child's foster home change, all information received by the previous foster home is provided to ensure continuity in the child's health care;

- involving the biological parents to the fullest extent possible in the child's health care; and

- providing the child's biological parents with information on the child's health status and needs, and helping them to plan for the child's health care when the child returns to them.

Health Care Rights

Children in foster care have the right to quality health care services that responds to their full range of needs. To ensure that children in foster care receive this high level of care, the foster parents and the caseworker who works with them have the right to:

- receive written, easy-to-understand information about the managed care plan;

- insist upon the availability of the range of services that are needed for the child;

- get answers from the child's doctor and/or plan representatives about the plan;

- get appointments for the child to see the health care provider within a reasonable period of time;

- have a choice of qualified health care providers for the child;

- receive understandable information about the child's health status;

- receive understandable information about the risks and benefits of the treatment the child is receiving;

- participate in decisions about the child's health care; and

- appeal decisions a plan makes about the child's care that do not appear to be in the child's best interests.

Chapter 5 presents, in question and answer format, typical concerns and problems that may arise in using managed care.

Advocacy Options

Managed care is a new system that can work well for children in foster car. In many instances, it has. Problems can arise, however, and foster parents and caseworkers should know what their options are.

Depending on the type of problem and the seriousness of the problem, a range of advocacy options are available. Foster parents and

> ### *Caseworker/Foster Parent Tip*
> The key to advocating for children in foster care is to ask questions and insist on answers. Don't be afraid to say that you do not understand or to insist on speaking to someone who can answer your questions.

caseworkers should work together as a team to decide which options are best under the circumstances. In all cases, the foster parents should let the caseworker and/or the supervisor know about the problems they are experiencing. Some of the options that foster parents and caseworkers can use are listed below.

1. Obtain a second opinion when there is a disagreement with the PCP. Ask to see another doctor who can give an opinion about what the child needs. Ask for a doctor who is experienced in working with children in foster care.

2. Appeal the decision of the plan.
Find out the plan's complaint and appeal procedures. Ask the plan service representative for any additional information that is needed and for assistance in complying with the procedures. Follow the procedures carefully. Be prepared to explain why the child needs the services that have been denied. Talk with others who know the child—teachers, neighbors, clergy—and ask them to write letters explaining why the child needs the denied services.

Find out how to proceed if the appeal is denied. Many plans have a grievance committee to review appeals that are denied. Some have several levels of appeals that can be used. Follow the plan's procedures carefully.

> ### *Caseworker/Foster Parent Tip*
> Appeals tend to take a long time—usually 30 to 90 days. Be prepared for a long process. Don't give up!

3. Call the Medicaid office for help.
Because managed care plans have contracts with the state Medicaid office, that office is interested in hearing from consumers regarding service provision. Ask to speak to the liaison between Medicaid and the managed care plan. The caseworker should help with this.

4. Contact consumer groups for help.
The problem may be one that other families are experiencing. Contact the Foster Parents Association, state advocacy groups for children, and/or organizations that focus on the needs of children in foster care for help.

5. Notify the court of the problem.
Courts may be able to take action if they become aware that a child in foster care is not receiving needed services.

6. Consult a lawyer.
A lawyer's advocacy may be helpful if attempting to work with the plan cooperatively fails and the child is still in need of services. In many states, a child in care has a lawyer and/or a court-appointed special advocate (CASA). The agency's attorney may also be able to help.

Chapter Five

Managed Care
Questions and Answers

Although each child's situation under managed care is unique, there are certain concerns common to all. The questions in this chapter are those most often raised by users of managed care. The answers provided are for general guidance only; in many instances, the answer can only be determined by checking the managed care organization's printed materials or benefit plan.

Who decides what care the child in our care needs?

The primary care physician (the PCP) decides whether care is "medically necessary"—that is, whether the child's medical condition requires it. It is important to know, however, whether the plan limits the PCP's options for treatment. Some plans provide doctors with a specific list of treatments that are approved for certain illnesses and conditions. Ask your PCP about your plan's rules.

What kind of limits should we expect on services?

Plans vary on the limits they put on services. Many plans require that certain procedures be done on an outpatient basis. Almost all plans limit the number of days a patient can stay in the hospital. It is also common for plans to limit mental health services either by limiting the number of visits the child can have with a mental health service provider or by limiting the amount of money that can be spent on mental health services. Home health services also may be limited. Check the written materials on your plan to see what limits the plan has. If the information is not clear, ask your PCP to explain the rules.

Do all services require prior approval?

No, but the majority do. Most hospital procedures and surgeries— whether done as outpatient or inpatient procedures—require prior approval. Other high-cost services—such as CT scans, MRIs, and specialists' services—usually also require prior approval. It is also common that plans require prior approval for mental health services, case management services, transportation, and specialty care, including care by pediatric specialists. Pediatric specialists are those doctors who are most knowledgeable about a child's particular health problem. For example, a pediatric cardiologist specializes in the heart problems of children. A pediatric ophthalmologist specializes in the eye problems of children. Check the written materials on your plan to find out what the plan's rules are on prior approvals. If the information is not clear, ask your PCP for help in understanding the rules.

If prior approval is required, how do we get it?

Your PCP will know what services require prior approval. Your PCP should be able to complete the necessary paperwork to obtain the prior approval. If your PCP cannot help with this process, you can contact the plan's office of customer relations. If necessary, discuss the matter immediately with your caseworker and/or his or her supervisor or the child welfare agency's health care coordinator.

When we met with our child's PCP for the first time, she hardly gave any time to examining him. When we tried to explain his background—that he is in foster care and that since coming to our home, he has been withdrawn and not sleeping well—she told us that she did not have time to get into a discussion and left before we could ask her what we should do to help the child. What options do we have?

It may be possible to talk with the PCP about the child and about her important role as the child's PCP. Try to work out the problem with her. Your caseworker should be kept informed every step of the way with any problems you experience. Find out from the plan's written materials or your caseworker the name and phone number of the plan's service representative. Call the representative and describe the problem. Keep a record of your conversation—the date of the call, the name of the representative, the information you provided, and the response you received. Ask the representative to explain your options and to tell you who you should contact as you follow the guidance he/ she gives you. If the representative is not helpful, follow the plan's written guidelines on filing a complaint.

We are concerned about our child's aggressive behavior toward other children in our home and asked our PCP if she could be evaluated by a mental health professional, but our PCP told us she would "grow out of it" and we shouldn't worry. We think it's more than just a phase. What should we do?

Ask for a second opinion. Talk with a plan service representative. Notify your caseworker or his/her supervisor immediately.

Can we see doctors and other health care providers not participating in the managed care plan?

It depends on your plan. Some plans allow services to be provided by doctors who are not in the plan's network, but usually, you must pay some portion of the doctor's fee. With other plans, if you go outside the provider network, you will need to pay the entire fee. Check the plan's written material to see what the policy is. You also can call the child welfare agency's health care coordinator or the managed care plan's office of customer relations.

Our PCP recommended that the child in our care undergo a series of allergy tests with a pediatric allergy specialist. He requested prior approval from the plan, but the request was denied. What options do we have if the plan refuses to authorize services the PCP recommends?

Obtain as much information as possible about who made the decision to deny services and how. Was it made by a medical review board or a single individual? Was the decision based on preset rules? Did the decision makers think that the test was not "medically necessary"? If so, how did they reach that decision? Ask your PCP to help you convince the decision makers that the tests are needed and explore the appeals process. Keep your caseworker informed and involved as much as possible.

Our PCP recommended that the child in our care see a pediatric cardiologist, but told us that there is no such specialist in the MCO provider network. What should we do?

Ask the PCP what the options are. Is it possible to go to a specialist outside the plan? Who would she recommend that your child see? Are there steps that the PCP can take in behalf of your child to get plan approval and payment for the child to see the needed specialist?

The child in our care needs ongoing mental health care services because she was severely physically abused. The plan says that a child can receive only eight mental health care visits a year. Our child has received the eight visits but it is obvious that she needs much more. What can we do?

Ask your PCP and/or the mental health care provider to request approval for an extension of services. If this request is denied, appeal the decision. Be sure to notify your caseworker and his/her supervisor immediately.

Will the doctor or plan remind us to come in for checkups?

It depends on your plan. Ask your doctor what the policy is. If the plan does not send reminders, mark your calendar to remind yourself of checkups.

Can we change the health plan of the child in our care?

Most plans allow for a change of plans at certain times during the year. This limitation can sometimes present a problem if the child moves to a new foster home. Discuss any problems with your caseworker. If you want to change plans because you are dissatisfied with the care your child is receiving, immediately discuss this problem with your caseworker and/or his supervisor.

What if the closest primary care provider is not easily accessible or far away. Can we get a PCP who is closer?

Again, check your plan policies. Talk with your caseworker and a plan representative. Find out if the plan or the agency can assist you with transportation services.

If our family is enrolled in a health plan, can the child in our care be in the same plan?

It may be possible to enroll your child in the same health care plan as the plan that you, as foster parents, use. Ask your caseworker if this is possible and if it is, in fact, the best plan for the child.

What if the child in our care gets sick late at night or on the weekend?

Almost all managed care plans have an after-hours number. Keep this number in a handy place and use it to receive advice over the phone or information on where to take the child to be seen. Be ready to give the person on the line your child's health insurance number and the name of your child's PCP.

What do we do in an emergency?

Medical emergencies are sudden, unexplained, or life-threatening situations that threaten the child's health or very severe illnesses or injuries that require immediate attention. Find out from your PCP, the plan's written materials, or a representative of the plan which hospitals are in the plan network and can be used in an emergency. If the child in your care is facing a life-threatening emergency, call an ambulance or take the child to the nearest hospital immediately.

Most plans have strict rules on using emergency rooms and will not pay for emergency room care unless it is a "true emergency." Whenever possible, call the managed care plan for directions on how to handle an emergency.

If it is a life-threatening emergency, go to the nearest hospital—a hospital in the plan network if possible.

What if we are out of town and the child in our care gets sick or hurt?

Most plans have rules about covering health care for emergencies when you are out of town. Most plans will cover "true emergencies" but will not cover routine or nonemergency care. Check your plan's written materials for these rules, and ask your PCP and/or caseworker for assistance if the information is not clear. When traveling out of town, always have with you the child's health care identification card and the telephone number for the plan in case of an emergency. If possible, call the plan before receiving services.

Will the child welfare agency pay for health care services not covered by the MCO?

The answer may depend on the policy of the child welfare agency and the type of service that is needed. Ask your caseworker for a written copy of the agency's policy.

Appendix A

Physical, Mental Health, and Developmental Concerns

Physical Concerns

Children in foster care often have chronic physical problems. Because these are long-term problems, they require special planning and services. The list that follows summarizes the symptoms of medical problems often present in children in care. It is not intended to replace diagnosis by a doctor or other health care professional.

Allergies
> Allergies are unusual reactions to everyday things like dust, certain foods, grass, medicines, or animals. The child's reactions can be severe or mild. Mild reactions can include itchy skin, a rash, runny eyes or nose, sneezing and wheezing, and stomachaches. Severe reactions may interfere with the child's ability to breath and can be life threatening.

Anemia/Iron Deficiency
> Anemia is a condition that occurs when the child does not have enough red blood cells. Iron deficiency means the child has too little iron in the blood. Children with these conditions may be pale, tired, or lack energy.

Asthma
> Children with asthma have difficulty breathing during asthma attacks. They may have a persistent dry cough, wheezing, or shortness of breath. Asthma attacks can be life threatening if not controlled and treated.

Dental Cavities/Problems with Teeth
> Cavities are tooth decay—that is, food and bacteria combine to attack the child's tooth enamel. The child may have tooth pain, missing teeth, or bad breath. Teeth that are overly crowded together or that stick out may affect the child's ability to eat and to speak.

Ear Infections/Hearing Problems
> Children who daydream, fail to follow directions, have poor balance, or don't speak well may have a hearing problem or ear infection. Children with ear infections may be symptomless or may have earaches, pus coming from the ears, or chronic tonsil infections.

Failure to Thrive
> Failure to thrive is a condition in which the child—usually an infant or toddler—does not grow or develop normally. The child may fail to gain weight or seem sad, cranky, or weak.

HIV Infection
> HIV is the virus that causes AIDS. The virus attacks the body's immune system and leaves the child likely to get many colds and serious infections. Children may be born HIV positive if their mothers have HIV, or may become infected through unprotected sexually activity or through intravenous drug use.

Malnutrition
> Malnutrition occurs when the child does not eat enough food or foods containing essential nutrients for normal physical growth. The child may look pale, thin, or wasted; have a bloated stomach; lack energy; appear sick or cranky; or have a poor attention span. Some children suffer from eating disorders that may include self-induced vomiting.

Musculoskeletal Problems

As children grow, their muscles develop and with them the children's ability to move around, grab things, sit, stand, etc. Some musculoskeletal problems are present from birth, such as a clubfoot. Others develop later in life, such as scoliosis (curvature of the spine). What appears to be a musculoskeletal problem, however, may be due to poor footwear or other apparel, or other injuries or illnesses, such as a fungus caused by poor hygiene.

Neurological Disabilities

Problems with the body's nervous system may show up in such symptoms as headaches, seizures, fainting, tremors, or problems with movement, coordination, and strength.

Poor Vision

Children who often stumble and fall, daydream, hold toys and books very close or very far away, or squint may have poor vision. Their difficulty in seeing makes their everyday activities difficult. Poor vision may also be associated with crossing of the eyes.

Sexually Transmitted Diseases (STD)

A wide variety of diseases can be transmitted through sexual contact. STDs may also be transmitted to an infant at the time of birth. STDs can cause no symptoms or can be life threatening. Children who have been sexually abused or youths who are sexually active should be screened for the presence of STDs.

Short Stature

Height is largely determined by family genes. During childhood, there are spurts or slow periods of growth and development. Long periods of no growth, however, can be a sign of illness.

Skin Problems

Skin problems can be caused by common childhood diseases like chicken pox; by insect bites, poison ivy, diaper rash, eczema, ringworm, or lice; by an allergic reaction (hives); or by emotional stress. The child's skin may itch, turn red, or develop spots, sores, oozing, or crustiness.

Mental Health Concerns

Children in care may have emotional problems as the result of abuse or neglect, separation from their biological families, a sense of uncertainty in their lives, or a combination of these factors. The list that follows summarizes the symptoms of mental health problems sometimes present in children in care. It is not intended to replace diagnosis by a doctor or other health care professional.

Anxiety
> The child who is anxious may be fearful, worried, or nervous.

Aggressiveness
> Fighting or threatening others, or cruelty to people or animals are signs of aggressive behavior.

Cognitive Difficulties
> A significant lessening in the ability to think or remember or understand may reflect a head injury or substance abuse.

Communication Difficulties
> Stuttering, difficulty expressing thoughts, or difficulty understanding others are among the most common communication problems.

Conduct Disorders
> Children who repeatedly and continually fight or are cruel to animals, or who steal, lie, or break rules, may have a conduct disorder.

Delinquency
> Delinquent behaviors can include stealing, destroying property, injuring others, and problems with the police.

Depression
> Children who are depressed may be very sad, tired, eat too little or too much, have trouble sleeping, or withdraw from activities.

Problems with Relationships/Attachment Disorders
　　The inability to develop friendships and other problems
　　children have getting along with family members, class-
　　mates, and/or teachers may reflect an emotional, mental, or
　　physical problem.

School Difficulties
　　Children learn at their own rate, but some problems can
　　interfere with their learning or their behavior in school.
　　Physical difficulties such as problems seeing, hearing, or
　　sleeping, or problems paying attention can cause children to
　　do poorly in school.

Self-Destructive Behaviors
　　Symptoms can include self-mutilation, suicide attempts,
　　running away, and acting out sexually.

Substance Abuse
　　A wide range of substances can be abused, including alcohol,
　　street drugs, over-the-counter medications, fuel, paint, and
　　glue. Symptoms of substance abuse include inattention,
　　social problems, poor school performance, and repeated
　　absences.

Developmental Concerns

Many children who are abused or neglected have developmental
problems. These problems range from mild sensory impairments
to severe physical disabilities. In some instances, a child's developmental problems may be the reason the child enters foster
care—the disability may make it extremely difficult for the biological parents to care for the child. The list that follows summarizes the symptoms of developmental problems often present in
children in care. It is not intended to replace diagnosis by a doctor
or other health care professional.

Attention Deficit Disorder
　　A child who makes many careless mistakes in schoolwork,
　　has trouble paying attention in class or activities, loses

things, is easily distracted, does not seem to listen, or is forgetful may have attention deficit disorder or attention deficit hyperactivity disorder.

Cerebral Palsy
Cerebral palsy may cause coordination problems of the arms, legs, or face. Children may have trouble controlling their muscles and may tremble, move stiffly, or slur their speech.

Delayed Growth and Development
A child may be slow to grow or to do things that are expected by a certain age. The child may take longer to walk, talk, or be toilet trained, or may have difficulty learning at school.

Learning Disabilities
A large difference between a child's intelligence and his or her school performance may indicate a learning disability. Schools are required by law to make accommodations for these problems if they interfere with the child's ability to learn.

Mental Retardation
Children learn at their own rate, but sometimes conditions caused by illness, accident, or problems experienced at birth can interfere with learning. The child may have trouble remembering information, following directions, or changing routines. The child may also be slow at learning or have trouble talking.

Appendix B

Managed Care Terminology

Access

The patient's ability to obtain medical care is often based on his or her ability to get to the doctor's office, to understand the language spoken by the doctor and staff, and to have the office open at convenient hours such as evenings, nights, and weekends

Behavioral Health Care

Psychological, psychiatric, and/or counseling services, including drug and alcohol abuse prevention and treatment programs, and services for mental health disorders

Capitation

A method of managed care reimbursement that pays doctors a fixed amount per patient, regardless of the amount or type of services the patient requires. Rather than charging for each service, MCOs receive a preset fee to meet an agreed-upon set of health care needs, and contract with doctors to provide services for a set fee. If the MCO's cost of providing services exceeds the prepaid fees, the MCO loses money. If the MCO's cost is less than the fees it charges, the MCO makes a profit.

Carve Out

Medicaid or others who contract for an MCO's services may tell the MCO not to offer certain services, such as dental care or mental health care, and may make arrangements for these services to be provided in other ways.

Fee for Service
The traditional model for health insurance in the United States, under which doctors provide a health care service, and bill the insurer, such as Medicaid, a set fee for that service.

Gatekeeper
The doctor or other health care provider who coordinates care and approves or disapproves care by specialists, hospital stays, or lab tests. Responsibility for "gatekeeping" is often shared with a "benefit reviewer" from the MCO.

Health Maintenance Organization (HMO)
A type of MCO that offers enrollees a selected group of providers who provide preventive services and medical care. Each patient's care is managed by one case manager or gatekeeper. HMOs require their enrollees to receive all of their care from within their plan's network.

- Staff model HMOs are usually nonprofit and have their own clinics, laboratories, and full-time salaried staffs.

- Network HMOs usually include providers who contract with the HMO to provide certain services.

Independent Practice Association (IPA)
A form of HMO that allows enrollees to see certain doctors in their own private offices, but requires that care be provided according to treatment, review, and approval protocols set by the plan. Enrollees are covered only when they use HMO-designated providers and hospitals.

Insurance
A system that pays for health care.

Managed Care
A form of health care that uses selective contracting as a means of channeling patients to a limited or set number of

providers. Managed care plans typically require a utilization review process to control what they deem to be unnecessary use of health services

Managed Care Organization (MCO)

An organization of health care providers, such as doctors and hospitals, formed to offer more efficient and less costly health care services.

Medicaid

A joint federal/state-financed program that purchases medical care services for low-income children, families, and the elderly. It is governed by a maze of federal and state laws, regulations, and guidelines. Because the Medicaid program is complex and costly to operate, governors in virtually every state are seeking to restructure the program.

Medical necessity

A standard that Medicaid uses as the test of whether a health care service is actually needed by a patient. While a certain service may be covered by Medicaid, the medical necessity standard provides Medicaid with a means for deciding—for a particular patient—what type of services will be provided and for how long they will be provided.

Because there is no definition of medical necessity, the standard is confusing and arbitrary in application. Usually, the primary care physician determines if a service is medically necessary, although a managed care plan may limit the doctor's options by a having a specific list of treatments that are approved for certain illnesses.

Point-of-Service Plan (POS)

A type of MCO that provides the bulk of services within an HMO and assigns enrollees to a primary care physician (gatekeeper). Enrollees may use services outside of the HMO, however, in exchange for paying a larger part of the cost.

Preferred Provider Organizations (PPO)

A type of MCO that offers enrollees a choice of certain doctors and hospitals within a community. PPO members may choose out-of-plan providers, but will be charged more for doing so.

Provider Network
> A group of health professionals or health care organizations that provides health care services to patients. Typically, a provider network has a central structure that cocrdinates services.

Special Health Care
> Health care services that are provided by medical specialists (such as surgeons or dermatologists) who generally are not the first doctors to see the patient.

Treatment Protocols
> The plan or steps to be followed in the care of a patient.

Appendix C
Sample Immunization Schedule

When Do Children and Teens Need Immunizations?*

Age	Immunization					
	Hepatitis B	Diphtheria/ Tetanus/ Pertussis	Haemophilus influenzae type b	Polio	Measles/ Mumps/ Rubella	Chickenpox
Birth	✓ (birth–2 months)[1]					
1 Month	✓ (1–4 months)[1]					
2 Months		✓	✓	✓		
4 Months		✓	✓	✓		
6 Months	✓ (6–18 months)[1]	✓	✓[2]			
12 Months			✓ (12–15 months)[1]	✓ (12–18 months)[1,3]	✓ (12–15 months)[1]	✓ (12–18 months)[1]

Age					
15 Months	✓ (12–18 months)[1,4]	✓	✓ (This is a Td shot. It does not contain pertussis vaccine.)		
4–6 Years		✓		✓ (Give at 4–6 years of age or at 11–12 years of age.)	
11–12 Years	✓✓✓ (All teens need 3 hepatitis B shots if they haven't already received them.)				Children who are 12 months of age through 12 years of age (who have not had chickenpox) need to be vaccinated with one dose.
13–16 Years					Children 13 years of age and older (who have not had chickenpox or been previously vaccinated) need 2 doses.

Were you or your child born in a country where hepatitis B is a common disease?

If so, your child, no matter what age, should be vaccinated against hepatitis B. Talk to your health care provider about whether your child needs to receive shots for hepatitis A, influenza, or pneumococcal disease. Certain children are at risk for these diseases and need to be immunized against them.

1. This is the age range in which the vaccine should be given.
2. Depending on the brand of vaccine used for the first and second doses, a dose at 6 months of age may not be needed.
3. If all oral polio vaccine is used, the third dose may be given as early as 6 months of age.
4. May be given as early as 12 months of age if 6 months of age have elapsed since the previous dose and if the child might not return by 18 months of age.

* Immunization chart provided courtesy of Immunization Action Coalition, St. Paul, MN.

Appendix D

The CWLA National Advisory Committee on Managed Health Care for Children in Foster Care

Bob Barker, M.S.W., Executive Director, Southwest Behavioral Healthcare Inc.

Steve Blatt, M.D., Director, Enhance Services for Children in Foster Care State University of New York Health Sciences Center

Fred Chaffee, Executive Director, Arizona Children's Home

Patrick Chaulk, M.D., Senior Associate, Annie E. Casey Foundation

Abigail English, J.D., Project Director, National Health Care Project, National Center for Youth Law

Harriette B. Fox, President, Fox Health Policy Consultants

Madelyn DeWoody Freundlich, J.D., M.S.W., M.S.P.H., Director, The Adoption Institute, Spence-Chapin Services to Families and Children

Neal Halfon, M.D., M.P.H., School of Public Health and Medicine, University of California

Lucille McCluney, Foster Parent, Branch Chief for Policy Review and Operations, U.S. Children's Bureau

Beatrice Moore, Deputy for Lashawn General Receivership, District of Columbia

Lavdena Orr, M.D., Director, Division of Child Protection, Children's National Medical Center
Monica Oss, President, OPEN MINDS, Inc.
Edward L. Schor, M.D., Medical Director, Division of Family and Community Health, Iowa Department of Public Health
Mark Simms, M.D., Director, Child Development Center, Children's Hospital of Wisconsin
Jake Terpstra, M.S.W., Licensing, Residential Care, and Child Welfare Specialist, U.S. Children's Bureau
Cleo Terry, M.S.W., Vice President, Child and Family Services, Lifelink Corporation/Bensenville Home Society
Kay Dean Toran, Director, State Office for Services to Children and Families, Oregon Department of Human Resources
Elizabeth Wehr, J.D., Center for Health Policy Research, George Washington University
Winifred Wilson, Director, Maryland Commission for Families

CWLA Staff

Kathy Barbell, Program Director, Family Foster Care
Ellen Battistelli, Senior Policy Analyst, Project Director
Charlotte McCullough, Director, Managed Care Institute
Karabelle Pizzigati, Director of Public Policy
Francine Ronis, Public Policy Assistant
Bruce Webb, Senior Consultant

About the Author

Ellen Sittenfeld Battistelli is Senior Health Policy Analyst for the Child Welfare League of America (CWLA), and Project Director for a Robert Wood Johnson Foundation grant to develop two guides on managed health care and children in foster care. She also oversees CWLA's participation in a Kaiser Family Foundation project on the impact of Medicaid on vulnerable populations. Prior to joining CWLA, she worked on public policy health issues as a Congressional staffer and as an analyst for national nonprofit organizations.

MAKING MANAGED HEALTH CARE WORK FOR KIDS IN FOSTER CARE
A Guide to Purchasing Services

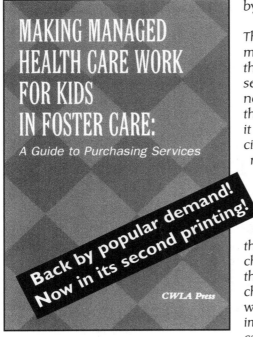

by Ellen Sittenfeld Battistelli

This guide can help purchasers of managed health care understand the complex health care and social service needs of an especially vulnerable population—children in the foster care system. In addition, it explains for child welfare agencies the goals and workings of managed health care.

Topics: What is foster care? Who are the children in foster care and how do they enter the system? Who is responsible for these children? What happens to children in foster care? What are the special health needs of these children? Sections also examine why comprehensive health care is important, Medicaid and managed care, implications for children in foster care, important issues and strategies for care, provider/managed care organization requirements, reimbursements, portability, access to services, confidentiality, benefit packages, specialized medical services, behavioral health care services, immediate eligibility, case management, record-keeping, quality assurance and quality improvement, prior approval, medical necessity, social necessity, state pressure to reduce Medicaid costs, and contract language.

A CWLA Press Publication.